Radiant Pregnancy

Maintaining a Balance with Exercise, Diet, and Mindfulness

Michael Murray

CONTENT

Chapter 1: Nurturing Life - The Foundations of Profound Pregnancy Wellness

Chapter 2: "The Foundations of Prenatal Wellness"

Chapter 3: Exercise for Radiance - Tailoring Wellness throughout Pregnancy

Chapter 4: Nutritional Foundations - Nourishing Body and Baby

Chapter 5: Mindfulness Practices for Expecting Mothers

Chapter 6: Holistic Self-Care Rituals - Nurturing the Body and Soul During Pregnancy

Chapter 7: Mindfulness Practices for Expecting Mothers

Chapter 8: Radiant Mind, Radiant Body - Exploring the Harmony of Mental and Physical Well-being during Pregnancy

Chapter 9: Partnering in Wellness - Strengthening Bonds through Shared Experiences.

Chapter 10: Continuing the Wellness Journey

Chapter 11: Radiant Mind, Radiant Body - Nurturing the Connection Between Mental and Physical Well-being

Chapter 12: Continuing the Wellness Journey - Sustaining Radiant Health Beyond Childbirth

INTRODUCTION

Embark on a journey of profound wellness during pregnancy, where we explore the concept of radiance, which encompasses physical, mental, and emotional well-being. Understanding the importance of balance sets the foundation for a radiant experience throughout the miraculous journey of pregnancy.

Nutritional Foundations: Nourish your body and your baby with essential nutrients by creating a well-rounded and nutrient-rich pregnancy diet. Dive into the importance of specific vitamins and minerals for fetal development while exploring delicious and nourishing meal options.

Exercise for Radiance: Tailor your exercise routines for different stages of pregnancy to promote overall well-being. From building foundations in the first trimester to mindful movements in the third, discover safe and effective workouts that enhance radiance and vitality.

Mindfulness Practices for Expecting Mothers: Cultivate a mindful mindset for a positive pregnancy experience. Explore techniques for managing stress, enhancing emotional well-being, and fostering a connection between mind and body during this transformative time.

Building a Supportive Environment: Surround yourself with a supportive network during pregnancy by communicating your needs and fostering a positive support system. Create an environment that encourages emotional well-being and provides the necessary support for this unique journey.

Profound Self-Care Rituals: Create a self-care routine that addresses both physical and emotional needs. Explore relaxation techniques and rituals that promote overall well-being, nurturing yourself in preparation for the incredible journey ahead.

Monitoring and Celebrating Milestones: Track the progress of your pregnancy journey, celebrating and embracing each stage of development. Reflect on the milestones, both big and small, as you nurture the growing connection with your baby.

Partnering in Wellness: Involve your partner in the wellness journey, strengthening your bond through shared experiences. Explore ways to enhance mutual support, understanding, and connection during this transformative time.

Radiant Mind, Radiant Body: Delve into the connection between mental and physical well-being. Explore mind-body techniques that promote radiant health, fostering a harmonious balance throughout your pregnancy.

Preparing for Labor and Delivery: Strategize for both mental and physical preparation for childbirth. Understand the birthing process and create a birth plan that aligns with your preferences, ensuring a more empowered and positive labor and delivery experience.

Postpartum Radiance: Transition into the postpartum period with grace, exploring postpartum self-care and recovery tips for a radiant new chapter. Navigate the challenges and joys of the early postpartum period with a focus on well-being.

Continuing the Wellness Journey: Integrate wellness practices into the post-pregnancy lifestyle, sustaining radiant health for both mother and baby beyond childbirth. Embrace the continuation of the wellness journey, adapting practices to suit the evolving needs of your growing family.

Chapter 1: Nurturing Life - The Foundations of Profound Pregnancy Wellness

Pregnancy is a transformative journey, and embracing a Profound approach to wellness is paramount for the well-being of both the expectant mother and the developing baby. This chapter delves into the foundational principles of Profound pregnancy wellness, exploring key elements that contribute to a healthy and thriving pregnancy experience.

Understanding ProfoundWellness:

Profound wellness in pregnancy goes beyond conventional medical care; it encompasses the integration of physical, mental, and emotional well-being. Recognizing that these aspects are interconnected is crucial for creating a supportive environment for both the mother and the growing life within.

Nutrition as the Cornerstone:
The expectant mother's diet plays a pivotal role in the baby's development and the overall health of both. For example, incorporating a variety of nutrient-dense foods, such as leafy greens, lean proteins, and whole grains, ensures a well-rounded supply of essential vitamins and minerals. Proper nutrition not only supports the baby's growth but also helps alleviate common pregnancy discomforts.

Exercise for Physical and Emotional Balance:

Physical activity is another key component. Regular, moderate exercise has been shown to enhance mood, reduce the risk of gestational diabetes, and improve overall fitness. Prenatal yoga, swimming, and brisk walking are excellent examples of low-impact exercises that can be adapted to various fitness levels. By incorporating movement into the daily routine, pregnant individuals can experience improved circulation, reduced stress, and enhanced muscle tone.

Embracing Mindfulness Practices:

Mindfulness is a powerful tool for navigating the emotional landscape of pregnancy. Techniques such as meditation, deep breathing, and guided imagery can help manage stress, anxiety, and mood swings. For instance, a simple daily mindfulness practice, focusing on the present moment and connecting with the baby, can foster a sense of calm and connection.

Creating a Supportive Environment:

Pregnancy wellness extends beyond individual practices to include the environment in which the expectant mother resides. Cultivating a supportive community, whether through prenatal classes, support groups, or connecting with other expectant parents, provides emotional support and valuable insights. Sharing experiences and information can help build confidence and resilience throughout the pregnancy journey.

Expert Insights:

To illustrate the practical application of these principles, let's consider the experience of a pregnant individual named Sarah. Sarah embraced a holistic approach to wellness by maintaining a balanced diet rich in prenatal vitamins and incorporating regular walks into her routine. She also attended prenatal yoga classes, which not only improved her physical well-being but also provided a space for mindfulness and relaxation.

Rita's journey exemplifies the interconnected nature of Profound pregnancy wellness. By nourishing her body with wholesome foods, staying active, and integrating mindfulness practices, she created a positive foundation for herself and her baby.

In conclusion, this chapter establishes the fundamental concepts of Profound pregnancy wellness. By focusing on nutrition, exercise, mindfulness, and creating a supportive environment, expectant mothers can lay the groundwork for a healthy and fulfilling pregnancy. The integration of these principles sets the stage for the chapters to come, which will delve deeper into specific aspects of Profound well-being for both mother and baby.

From nutrition to exercise and emotional well-being, establishing a strong foundation during pregnancy is crucial for the health and development of both the mother and the baby.

Nutrition: The Cornerstone of Prenatal Health

One of the cornerstones of a healthy pregnancy is proper nutrition. During this transformative period, the body undergoes significant changes, necessitating an increased intake of essential nutrients. For example, folic acid is vital in preventing neural tube defects, and iron is crucial for preventing anemia. Including a variety of nutrient-dense foods, such as leafy greens, lean proteins, and whole grains, provides the necessary building blocks for a thriving pregnancy.

Example: Incorporating a colorful array of fruits and vegetables not only adds flavor to meals but also ensures a diverse range of vitamins and minerals essential for fetal development.

Exercise: Energizing the Journey

Contrary to outdated beliefs, exercise is not only safe but highly beneficial during pregnancy. Moderate, regular physical activity can alleviate common discomforts like back pain, boost mood, and promote better sleep. From brisk walking to prenatal yoga, tailored exercise routines can enhance cardiovascular health and maintain a healthy weight, contributing to an overall sense of well-being.

Example: A 30-minute daily walk not only supports cardiovascular health but also provides a low-impact way to stay active throughout pregnancy.

Emotional Well-Being: Nurturing the Mind and Spirit

Pregnancy is not only a physical journey but an emotional one as well. Addressing the psychological aspect of well-being is paramount for a positive pregnancy experience. Practices such as mindfulness meditation, deep-breathing exercises, and seeking emotional support can help manage stress and anxiety, fostering a serene environment for the growing baby.

Example: Mindful breathing exercises, like the 4-7-8 technique, can be integrated into daily routines to promote relaxation and reduce stress levels.

Integrating Wellness Practices: A Holistic Approach

This Chapter emphasizes the importance of integrating these foundational elements into a holistic approach to prenatal wellness. It's not about isolated actions but rather a synergistic combination of nutrition, exercise, and emotional well-being that creates a robust foundation for a healthy pregnancy.

Example: Combining a nutrient-rich meal with a gentle prenatal yoga session and a few moments of mindful reflection can create a comprehensive approach to daily prenatal care.

Expert Insights: Guiding the Journey

Throughout the chapter, expert insights are interwoven to provide evidence-based guidance. Health professionals, including obstetricians, nutritionists, and fitness specialists, contribute their expertise to ensure that the reader receives accurate and reliable information. This collaborative approach ensures that the foundations of prenatal wellness are not only understood but also personalized to meet individual needs.

In conclusion, This chapter establishes the pillars of prenatal wellness, laying the groundwork for a healthy and fulfilling pregnancy journey. By embracing nutrition, exercise, and emotional well-being in a holistic manner, expectant mothers can navigate this transformative period with confidence and grace. The chapter sets the stage for the subsequent exploration of specific wellness practices, offering a roadmap for nurturing both body and spirit during the incredible journey of pregnancy.

Chapter 3: Exercise for Radiance - Tailoring Wellness throughout Pregnancy

Exercise during pregnancy is a key component of maintaining overall well-being for both the mother and baby. In this chapter, we delve into the importance of incorporating safe and effective workouts at different stages of pregnancy. The goal is to not only support physical health but also enhance the radiance and vitality of expectant mothers.

Understanding Exercise for Radiance:

Exercise during pregnancy is often approached with caution, but when done correctly, it can contribute significantly to a woman's well-being. The term "radiance" here encompasses not just physical health but also the positive impact on mental and emotional states. Engaging in appropriate exercise routines can boost energy levels, alleviate mood swings, and improve overall self-esteem.

Tailoring Exercise Routines for Different Stages:

Pregnancy is a dynamic process, and the exercise routine should adapt accordingly. Let's explore how exercise can be tailored for each trimester:

• First Trimester: Foundations of Wellness

• Focus on low-impact activities like walking, swimming, or prenatal yoga to establish a foundation.

• Example: Morning walks provide a gentle cardiovascular workout while promoting a positive mindset.

• Second Trimester: Embracing Strength and Balance

• Incorporate strength training exercises with a focus on maintaining good posture and balance.

• Example: Bodyweight squats and modified lunges strengthen the lower body while enhancing stability.

• Third Trimester: Mindful Movement and Preparation

• Emphasize gentle movements and stretches to ease discomfort and prepare for labor.

• Example: Prenatal Pilates helps maintain flexibility and encourages mindful breathing.

Incorporating Safe and Effective Workouts:

Safety is paramount when designing exercise routines for pregnant women. Consider the following principles:

• Consultation with Healthcare Provider:

• Always consult with a healthcare provider before starting or modifying an exercise routine during pregnancy.

• Example: If there are any complications or specific health concerns, a healthcare provider may recommend modifications or specific exercises to avoid.

• Listen to Your Body:

• Pay attention to how your body responds to exercise and modify intensity or activities accordingly.

• Example: If a particular movement causes discomfort, find alternative exercises that achieve similar benefits.

• Hydration and Temperature Regulation:

• Stay well-hydrated and avoid overheating during exercise sessions.

• Example: Opt for indoor workouts or early morning/evening sessions to avoid extreme temperatures.

• Pelvic Floor Exercises:

• Include exercises to strengthen the pelvic floor, which can be particularly beneficial during and after pregnancy.

• Example: Kegel exercises help maintain pelvic floor health and can contribute to a smoother recovery postpartum.

Conclusion:

Exercise for radiance during pregnancy involves a thoughtful and adaptable approach to support the changing needs of the body. By tailoring exercise routines for different stages and incorporating safe practices, expectant mothers can nurture their physical, mental, and emotional well-being. Remember, the goal is not only to stay active but to cultivate a radiant and positive experience throughout the incredible journey of pregnancy.

Pregnancy is a transformative period, demanding careful attention to nutritional needs for both the mother's well-being and the optimal development of the growing baby. In this chapter, we delve into the nutritional foundations of a radiant pregnancy, exploring the importance of essential nutrients, creating a well-rounded pregnancy diet, and ensuring a wholesome approach to nourishment.

Importance of Essential Nutrients:

The foundation of a healthy pregnancy lies in providing the necessary nutrients crucial for fetal development and maternal well-being. Examples of key nutrients include:

• Folic Acid: is essential for neural development and is found in leafy greens, legumes, and fortified cereals.

• Calcium: is vital for bone development and is found in dairy products, fortified plant-based milk, and leafy greens.

• Iron: supports increased blood volume and is found in lean meats, beans, and fortified cereals.

• Omega-3 Fatty Acids: Important for brain and vision development, found in fatty fish, flaxseeds, and walnuts.

• Protein: is crucial for tissue development and is found in lean meats, eggs, dairy, and plant-based sources like legumes.

• Vitamin D: Aids in calcium absorption, found in fatty fish, fortified dairy, and exposure to sunlight.

Understanding these nutrients and their sources ensures a comprehensive approach to prenatal nutrition, promoting a healthy pregnancy.

Creating a Well-Rounded Pregnancy Diet:

A well-rounded pregnancy diet involves incorporating a variety of nutrient-dense foods to meet increased energy and nutritional needs. Examples of a balanced pregnancy diet include:

• Fruits and Vegetables: Provide essential vitamins, minerals, and fiber. Aim for a colorful array to maximize nutrient intake.

• Whole Grains: Rich in fiber and energy, examples include whole wheat, quinoa, and brown rice.

• Lean Proteins: Essential for tissue development and repair. Include sources like poultry, fish, tofu, and legumes.

• Dairy or Dairy Alternatives: Ensure an adequate intake of calcium for bone development. Opt for fortified plant-based milk if lactose intolerant.

• Healthy Fats: Incorporate sources like avocados, nuts, and olive oil for essential fatty acids.

• Hydration: Drink plenty of water to support increased blood volume and amniotic fluid.

Examples of Nutrient-Rich Meals:

• Quinoa Salad with Leafy Greens and Grilled Chicken:

• Packed with protein, iron, and fiber, this meal supports energy levels and essential nutrient intake.

• Salmon with Roasted Vegetables:

• Rich in omega-3 fatty acids and a variety of vitamins from colorful vegetables, it promotes overall fetal development.

• Greek Yogurt Parfait with Berries and Granola:

• Provides calcium, protein, and antioxidants, supporting bone development and overall maternal health.

• Lentil and Vegetable Stir-Fry:

• A plant-based option rich in iron, folate, and protein, catering to various nutritional needs during pregnancy.

Adapting the Diet for Individual Needs:

Individual nutritional needs vary, and adaptations may be necessary based on factors like dietary preferences, allergies, or medical conditions. Consulting with a healthcare provider or a registered dietitian ensures personalized guidance and support.

In conclusion, the nutritional foundations of a radiant pregnancy involve a thoughtful and diverse approach to food choices. By understanding the importance of essential nutrients, creating a well-rounded pregnancy diet, and adapting to individual needs, expectant mothers can nourish both their bodies and their growing babies, laying the groundwork for a healthy and vibrant pregnancy journey.

Chapter 5: Mindfulness Practices for Expecting Mothers

Mindfulness is a powerful tool that can significantly enhance the pregnancy experience by fostering a deep connection between mind and body. In this chapter, we delve into various mindfulness practices tailored for expecting mothers, offering techniques to manage stress, enhance emotional well-being, and cultivate a positive mindset throughout the transformative journey of pregnancy.

Understanding the Importance of Mindfulness:

Mindfulness involves being fully present in the current moment and acknowledging and accepting one's thoughts and feelings without judgment. During pregnancy, practicing mindfulness can have profound effects on mental and emotional well-being.

It provides a space for expectant mothers to connect with the changes happening within their bodies and to build a strong foundation for the challenges and joys of motherhood.

Techniques for Managing Stress:

Pregnancy often comes with its share of stress and anxiety. Mindfulness practices offer effective ways to manage these challenges, promoting a sense of calm and resilience. Deep breathing exercises, such as diaphragmatic breathing or progressive muscle relaxation, can be powerful tools. For example, taking slow, intentional breaths during moments of stress activates the body's relaxation response, reducing tension and promoting a sense of calm.

Enhancing Emotional Well-Being:

Emotional well-being is crucial during pregnancy, and mindfulness practices provide a toolkit for navigating the emotional highs and lows. Journaling is one such practice, allowing expectant mothers to express their thoughts and feelings freely. By acknowledging and processing emotions through writing, women can gain clarity and cultivate a positive emotional state. Reflective prompts, such as "What am I grateful for today?" or "How am I feeling physically and emotionally?" can guide this mindful journaling process.

Cultivating a Mindful Mindset:

Cultivating a mindful mindset involves bringing awareness to daily activities and fostering a non-judgmental awareness of one's thoughts and feelings. Meditation is a powerful tool for this purpose. Guided mindfulness meditations tailored for pregnancy, focusing on the breath or body sensations, can help mothers develop a deeper connection with their changing bodies and growing babies. For instance, a brief meditation where the expectant mother visualizes a warm, glowing light surrounding her and her baby can evoke a sense of calm and connection.

Incorporating Mindfulness into Everyday Life:

Practicing mindfulness doesn't always require a dedicated meditation session. Simple activities can be infused with mindfulness, promoting a sense of presence and connection. Mindful walking, for example, involves paying attention to each step, feeling the ground beneath the feet, and observing the surroundings. This practice not only provides physical activity but also serves as a mindfulness exercise, grounding the expectant mother in the present moment.

Guidance for Techniques and Resources:

Offering guidance on various mindfulness techniques, including meditation, mindful breathing, and mindful movement, equips expecting mothers with a diverse set of tools. Additionally, recommending reputable resources, such as mindfulness apps tailored for pregnancy or local prenatal yoga classes, ensures accessibility and ongoing support.

In conclusion, this chapter emphasizes the transformative impact of mindfulness practices on the pregnancy journey. By embracing mindfulness, expectant mothers can navigate stress, enhance emotional well-being, and cultivate a positive mindset. The incorporation of practical techniques and examples empowers mothers to integrate mindfulness into their daily lives, fostering a deeper connection with themselves and their growing babies.

Chapter 6: Holistic Self-Care Rituals - Nurturing the Body and Soul During Pregnancy

Pregnancy is a transformative journey that demands a holistic approach to self-care. This chapter delves into the essential concept of holistic self-care rituals, emphasizing the importance of nurturing both the body and soul during this remarkable period.

Creating a Self-Care Routine: Holistic self-care involves intentionally addressing physical and emotional needs. Begin by creating a self-care routine tailored to your preferences and lifestyle. This routine can include activities that bring joy, relaxation, and a sense of connection with your changing body.

Example: Incorporating a daily ritual, such as a warm bath infused with soothing essential oils, provides a calming space for self-reflection and relaxation.

Physical Well-Being: Nurturing the body is a central aspect of holistic self-care during pregnancy. This includes maintaining regular exercise, prioritizing adequate sleep, and paying attention to nutritional needs. Physical well-being contributes not only to the health of the mother but also to the optimal development of the growing baby.

Example: Engaging in prenatal yoga or gentle stretching exercises promotes flexibility, reduces tension, and fosters a connection between the body and mind.

Emotional Well-Being: Pregnancy brings forth a range of emotions, and tending to your emotional well-being is vital. Explore mindfulness practices, journaling, or engaging in activities that bring joy and tranquility. Emotional well-being plays a crucial role in creating a positive and harmonious environment for both you and your baby.

Example: Practicing daily gratitude by keeping a gratitude journal helps shift focus to positive aspects, fostering emotional well-being.

Incorporating Relaxation Techniques: Holistic self-care rituals often involve relaxation techniques to alleviate stress and promote a sense of calm. Deep-breathing exercises, meditation, or guided imagery can be integrated into your routine to create moments of tranquility amid the busyness of pregnancy.

Example: A five-minute deep-breathing exercise before bedtime can improve sleep quality and induce a sense of relaxation, contributing to overall well-being.

Mindful Eating: Nourishing your body with a well-balanced and nutrient-rich diet is a fundamental aspect of holistic self-care. Mindful eating involves paying attention to hunger and fullness cues, making conscious food choices, and savoring each bite. This approach supports not only physical health but also a positive relationship with food during pregnancy.

Example: Creating a colorful and diverse plate with a variety of fruits, vegetables, and whole grains ensures a nutrient-rich diet that benefits both mother and baby.

Balancing Rest and Activity: Holistic self-care recognizes the importance of balance between rest and activity. While staying physically active is crucial, allowing the body sufficient rest is equally vital. Listen to your body's cues, adjust activities accordingly, and ensure you allocate time for restorative practices.

Example: A balance between a morning walk for physical activity and an afternoon nap for rest helps maintain energy levels and overall well-being.

Reflection and Connection: Incorporate moments of reflection into your self-care routine to connect with the profound experience of pregnancy. This can involve keeping a pregnancy journal, engaging in visualization exercises, or simply spending quiet moments acknowledging the miraculous journey you are undertaking.

Example: Setting aside time each week for a quiet reflection session, where you connect with your growing baby, can enhance the sense of bonding and mindfulness.

In conclusion, Chapter 6 guides expecting mothers through the intricacies of holistic self-care rituals, emphasizing the significance of nurturing both the body and soul during pregnancy. By incorporating personalized self-care routines, addressing physical and emotional well-being, and integrating relaxation techniques, mothers can cultivate a radiant and positive pregnancy experience.

Chapter 7: Mindfulness Practices for Expecting Mothers

Mindfulness during pregnancy is a transformative practice that goes beyond the physical aspects of well-being, delving into the realm of mental and emotional health. This chapter explores the importance of cultivating a mindful mindset for a positive pregnancy experience, provides techniques for managing stress, and enhancing overall emotional well-being.

Understanding Mindfulness in Pregnancy: Mindfulness is the practice of being fully present in the current moment without judgment. When applied to pregnancy, it involves embracing the physical and emotional changes with awareness and acceptance. This practice empowers expecting mothers to navigate the challenges and joys of pregnancy with a sense of calm and resilience.

Techniques for Managing Stress: Pregnancy often comes with a range of stressors, from physical discomfort to concerns about the future. Mindfulness techniques can serve as powerful tools for managing stress. One effective method is mindful breathing, where you focus on your breath to center yourself in the present moment. For example, taking a few minutes each day to engage in deep, intentional breaths can help alleviate stress and promote a sense of calm.

Enhancing Emotional Well-Being: Emotional well-being is a crucial aspect of a positive pregnancy experience. Mindfulness practices contribute to emotional balance by encouraging self-awareness and self-compassion. Journaling is one example of a mindfulness practice that promotes emotional well-being. By expressing thoughts and feelings on paper, expecting mothers can gain clarity, process emotions, and foster a deeper connection with their inner selves.

Mindful Movement for Pregnancy: Mindfulness extends to physical activity, incorporating gentle movements and exercises that promote a mind-body connection. Prenatal yoga is an excellent example of mindful movement. It combines gentle poses with intentional breathing, fostering flexibility, strength, and mental focus. Practicing prenatal yoga regularly not only supports physical health but also provides a space for expecting mothers to connect with their bodies and their growing babies.

Mindful Eating for Two: Nutrition is a key component of a healthy pregnancy, and mindfulness can be applied to eating habits. Mindful eating involves savoring each bite, paying attention to hunger and fullness cues, and being aware of the nutritional value of food. An example of mindful eating during pregnancy is taking the time to appreciate the flavors and textures of nutritious meals, fostering a positive relationship with food and nourishing both the mother and the baby.

Building Resilience Through Mindfulness: Pregnancy brings both anticipated and unexpected challenges. Mindfulness practices build resilience by encouraging a non-judgmental awareness of thoughts and feelings. Loving-kindness meditation is one way to cultivate resilience. This practice involves extending positive thoughts and wishes to oneself and others, fostering a sense of compassion and strength in the face of challenges.

Mindfulness in Everyday Activities: Being mindful doesn't always require a formal practice. Simple, everyday activities can become opportunities for mindfulness. For instance, washing dishes or taking a leisurely walk can be transformed into mindful moments by fully engaging in the experience, using the senses to appreciate the present.

Conclusion: Mindfulness is not just a technique; it's a way of living during pregnancy. By incorporating mindfulness practices into daily life, expecting mothers can create a positive and enriching experience. From managing stress to enhancing emotional well-being, mindfulness becomes a guiding light, fostering a deep connection with oneself and the miraculous journey of pregnancy.

Chapter 8: Radiant Mind, Radiant Body - Exploring the Harmony of Mental and Physical Well-being during Pregnancy

Understanding the Connection: The mind and body are intertwined, each influencing the other in profound ways. During pregnancy, this connection becomes even more pronounced, impacting the well-being of both the expectant mother and her growing baby. A radiant mind contributes to a positive physical experience, while a healthy body supports mental resilience.

Mind-Body Techniques for Radiant Health: In this chapter, we dive into mind-body techniques that promote radiant health during pregnancy. One notable example is mindfulness meditation. This practice involves bringing awareness to the present moment, reducing stress, and fostering a sense of calm. Through mindful breathing and guided meditation, expectant mothers can create a harmonious balance between their mental and physical states.

Example: Mindful Breathing Exercise

• Find a quiet space, sit comfortably, and close your eyes.

• Inhale deeply, counting to four, allowing your belly to expand.

• Exhale slowly, counting to six, releasing any tension.

• Repeat this process, focusing on your breath and bringing attention to the present moment.

Nurturing Mental Resilience: Pregnancy often comes with a range of emotions, from excitement to anxiety. Cultivating mental resilience is crucial for navigating these emotional landscapes. Practices such as positive affirmations and visualization exercises can empower expectant mothers, fostering a positive mindset.

Example: Positive Affirmations

• Create a list of affirmations that resonate with you.

• Repeat these affirmations daily to reinforce positive thoughts.

• Examples: "I trust my body's ability to nurture and grow my baby," or "I am resilient and capable of embracing each stage of my pregnancy with grace."

Addressing Stress and Anxiety: Pregnancy can bring about heightened stress and anxiety, impacting both mental and physical well-being. Chapter 8 explores various techniques for managing stress, including progressive muscle relaxation, guided imagery, and journaling. By acknowledging and addressing stressors, expectant mothers can foster a more serene and balanced mental state.

Example: Guided Imagery

• Find a quiet space and close your eyes.

• Imagine a peaceful scene, such as a tranquil beach or a serene forest.

• Engage your senses by visualizing the surroundings, feeling the warmth of the sun, or the gentle breeze.

• Allow this mental escape to promote relaxation and reduce stress.

The Role of Exercise in Mental Well-being: Physical activity is not only beneficial for the body but also plays a pivotal role in enhancing mental well-being.

Regular, moderate exercise releases endorphins, which are natural mood lifters. Yoga, in particular, combines physical movement with mindfulness, offering a holistic approach to both mental and physical fitness during pregnancy.

Example: Prenatal Yoga

• Engage in a prenatal yoga class that focuses on gentle movements and mindful breathing.

• Poses like the cat-cow stretch and child's pose can promote relaxation and alleviate tension.

• Connect with your breath, fostering a sense of tranquility throughout the practice.

Creating a Radiant Experience: this chapter concludes by emphasizing the importance of integrating these mind-body techniques into daily life. By consistently incorporating practices that nurture both the mind and body, expectant mothers can enhance their overall well-being, fostering a radiant experience throughout pregnancy.

In essence, it serves as a guide to unlocking the synergy between mental and physical well-being, empowering expectant mothers to embrace the transformative journey with resilience, positivity, and a radiant spirit.

Chapter 9: Partnering in Wellness - Strengthening Bonds through Shared Experiences.

Welcoming a new life into the world is not just a journey for the expectant mother but a transformative experience for partners as well. In this chapter, we explore the significance of involving your partner in the wellness journey during pregnancy, fostering a deeper connection and mutual support.

Creating Shared Experiences:

Pregnancy is a shared experience that extends beyond the expectant mother. Partners play a crucial role in creating a supportive and nurturing environment. Engaging in shared experiences, such as attending prenatal classes together, going for walks, or participating in birthing preparation workshops, strengthens the emotional bond and reinforces a sense of togetherness.

Example: Couples can join childbirth education classes where they learn about labor, delivery, and postpartum care together. This shared knowledge empowers both partners and fosters a collaborative approach to the upcoming changes.

Understanding Each Other's Perspectives:

Pregnancy brings forth a multitude of emotions and physical changes. Partners can deepen their connection by taking the time to understand each other's perspectives. Open and empathetic communication allows both individuals to express their concerns, expectations, and excitement, creating a foundation of mutual understanding.

Example: Setting aside dedicated time for open conversations about expectations and fears can enhance emotional intimacy. This shared understanding provides a strong base for navigating the challenges and joys of pregnancy together.

Active Participation in Wellness Practices:

Wellness during pregnancy extends beyond medical appointments and involves lifestyle choices. Partners can actively participate in wellness practices by adopting healthy habits together. From preparing nutritious meals to engaging in gentle exercises, shared wellness activities contribute to a supportive and health-focused household.

Example: Cooking nutritious meals together not only supports the expectant mother's dietary needs but also encourages a collaborative and enjoyable experience. It becomes a shared responsibility that reinforces the importance of health for both partners.

Attending Medical Appointments Together:

Being present at medical appointments is a tangible way for partners to actively participate in the pregnancy journey. Attending ultrasounds, check-ups, and important milestones together enhances the sense of shared responsibility and connection with the growing baby.

Example: Witnessing the ultrasound together can be a profound experience. Seeing the baby's development on the screen and hearing the heartbeat creates a shared moment of awe and joy, strengthening the emotional bond.

Providing Emotional Support:

Pregnancy can bring about a range of emotions for both partners. Providing emotional support becomes paramount during times of uncertainty or stress. Partners can offer a listening ear, express empathy, and actively participate in stress-reducing activities to create a positive emotional environment.

Example: Engaging in mindfulness practices together, such as deep breathing or meditation, can be a shared emotional outlet. These practices not only reduce stress but also create a calming atmosphere for both partners.

Preparing for the Transition to Parenthood:

Anticipating the arrival of a baby involves preparing not only for the birth but also for the transition to parenthood. Partners can attend parenting classes, read parenting books together, and discuss their roles and expectations, fostering a united front as they navigate the exciting yet challenging journey ahead.

Example: Taking part in a parenting class that covers topics like baby care, breastfeeding, and postpartum adjustment provides partners with practical knowledge and strengthens their readiness for parenthood.

In conclusion, this chapter emphasizes the importance of partnering in wellness during pregnancy. By actively involving partners in shared experiences, understanding each other's perspectives, and participating in wellness practices together, couples can strengthen their emotional connection and create a supportive foundation for the transformative journey into parenthood.

Chapter 10: Continuing the Wellness Journey

The culmination of pregnancy doesn't mark the end but rather the beginning of a new chapter—the post-pregnancy lifestyle. Chapter 10 is a guide to seamlessly integrating wellness practices into this evolving journey, ensuring sustained radiant health for both mother and baby beyond childbirth.

Integrating Wellness Practices: As the demands of motherhood unfold, integrating wellness practices becomes paramount. This involves adapting self-care routines, exercise regimens, and nutritional habits to align with the evolving needs of a growing family. For instance, continue to prioritize nutrient-rich meals while considering the time constraints of caring for a newborn.

Nurturing a Growing Family: The wellness journey extends to nurturing a growing family, fostering an environment that prioritizes health and well-being for everyone. This may involve incorporating family-friendly activities that encourage physical activity, such as nature walks or playful exercises that involve the little ones.

Adapting Self-Care Rituals: Self-care rituals established during pregnancy need adaptation to suit the demands of postpartum life. Integrating shorter, targeted self-care activities into daily routines, such as quick mindfulness exercises or brief moments of relaxation, allows for the continuation of nurturing one's mental and emotional well-being.

Postpartum Exercise and Recovery: Chapter 10 guides new mothers through postpartum exercise and recovery, emphasizing gradual reintegration of physical activity. Gentle exercises like postnatal yoga or walking contribute to both physical recovery and mental well-being. This adaptation ensures a safe transition back into an active lifestyle.

Embracing Change with Mindfulness: Mindfulness practices become even more crucial in navigating the challenges of early parenthood. Being present in the moment, whether soothing a crying baby or savoring precious quiet moments, contributes to a positive and resilient mindset. Mindfulness also aids in managing the inevitable changes and uncertainties that accompany parenting.

Prioritizing Sleep and Rest: Quality sleep is a cornerstone of overall wellness. Chapter 10 emphasizes the importance of prioritizing sleep and rest, offering practical tips for new parents to optimize their sleep patterns. Creating a conducive sleep environment and establishing a consistent bedtime routine contribute to the rejuvenation necessary for the demands of parenting.

Balancing Work and Family Life: For mothers returning to work, finding a balance between professional commitments and family life is a key consideration. It explores strategies for maintaining this delicate equilibrium, including effective time management, setting boundaries, and seeking support from both workplace and family.

Sustaining Nutritional Wellness: Nutritional wellness remains a focal point in post-pregnancy life. Continuing to nourish the body with nutrient-dense foods supports energy levels, overall health, and, if applicable, breastfeeding. Practical examples include creating meal plans that accommodate a busy schedule and choosing convenient yet nutritious snacks.

Celebrating Parenting Milestones: Just as pregnancy milestones were celebrated, it encourages the celebration of parenting milestones. Whether it's a baby's first smile, the first steps, or reaching developmental milestones, taking the time to acknowledge and celebrate these moments contributes to a positive and joyful parenting experience.

Maintaining Connection with Partner: The wellness journey extends to the relationship with a partner. Nurturing the connection through open communication, shared responsibilities, and quality time together strengthens the foundation of the family unit. Engaging in activities that foster bonding, such as date nights or collaborative parenting strategies, contributes to a supportive and harmonious partnership.

In essence, Chapter 10 encapsulates the ongoing nature of the wellness journey, acknowledging that the path to radiant health extends beyond pregnancy. By adapting practices, embracing change with mindfulness, and prioritizing the well-being of both mother and baby, this chapter serves as a guide to thriving in the dynamic landscape of parenthood.

In this transformative journey of pregnancy, we shall focus on the symbiotic relationship between the mind and body. this chapter explores the profound impact that mental well-being can have on physical health and vice versa, offering insights and practical techniques to cultivate a harmonious balance.

Understanding the Connection:

The mind and body are intricately connected, and this connection is particularly significant during pregnancy. A radiant mind contributes to a radiant body, promoting overall health and vitality for both the expectant mother and her developing baby. Conversely, physical well-being positively influences mental states, creating a holistic approach to pregnancy wellness.

Mind-Body Techniques for Promoting Radiant Health:

• Mindful Breathing:

• Example: Introduce deep-breathing exercises to alleviate stress and promote relaxation. Inhale slowly, allowing the abdomen to expand, then exhale gently, releasing tension.

• Yoga and Meditation:

• Example: Incorporate prenatal yoga and meditation practices to enhance flexibility, reduce anxiety, and foster a calm and centered mind.

Visualization Techniques:

• Example: Guide expectant mothers through positive visualization, helping them envision a smooth pregnancy journey and a positive birthing experience.

Affirmations for Positivity:

• Example: Encourage the use of affirmations that promote confidence and optimism, reinforcing a positive mindset throughout the pregnancy.

The Impact of Stress on Pregnancy:

High stress levels during pregnancy can have adverse effects on both the mother and the baby. Chronic stress may contribute to complications such as preterm birth and low birth weight. Therefore, managing stress becomes a crucial aspect of promoting a radiant mind and body.

Strategies for Stress Management:

• Mindfulness Meditation:

• Example: Introduce brief mindfulness meditation sessions to help expectant mothers stay present and manage stress effectively.

• Progressive Muscle Relaxation:

• Example: Teach progressive muscle relaxation techniques, guiding individuals to systematically tense and then release different muscle groups to reduce physical and mental tension.

• Expressive Writing:

• Example: Suggest the practice of expressive writing, where expectant mothers journal their thoughts and emotions as a therapeutic outlet for stress relief.

The Power of Positive Thinking:

Cultivating a positive mindset can significantly contribute to a radiant pregnancy experience. Positive thinking not only influences mental well-being but also supports physical health, creating a cycle of well-being.

Practical Techniques for Fostering Positivity:

• Gratitude Journaling:

• Example: Recommend keeping a gratitude journal to focus on positive aspects, fostering a sense of appreciation and joy.

• Mindful Appreciation:

• Example: Encourage moments of mindful appreciation, where expectant mothers take time to savor positive experiences and cultivate a sense of gratitude.

Creating a Supportive Mindset for Labor and Delivery:

The mindset cultivated during pregnancy can significantly impact the experience of labor and delivery. By preparing the mind for the challenges and joys of childbirth, expectant mothers can approach this transformative event with confidence and resilience.

Visualization for Positive Birth Experience:

• Example: Guide expectant mothers in visualizing a positive birth experience, helping them build confidence in their ability to navigate the birthing process.

In conclusion, this chapter emphasizes the importance of nurturing the connection between the mind and body for a radiant pregnancy. By incorporating mind-body techniques, managing stress effectively, and fostering a positive mindset, expectant mothers can enhance their overall well-being, creating a foundation for a healthy and harmonious pregnancy journey.

Integrating Wellness Practices: The journey of wellness doesn't end with childbirth; it evolves. Integrating wellness practices into your post-pregnancy lifestyle is vital for sustained well-being. This involves adapting to the new demands of motherhood while prioritizing self-care. For example, a postpartum yoga routine can provide both physical exercise and moments of mindfulness amidst the demands of a new baby.

Embracing Adaptation: Motherhood is a transformative experience, and adapting to the changes is key to maintaining radiant health. Recognizing that your wellness routine might need adjustments as your baby grows and your schedule changes allows for a more flexible and sustainable approach. For instance, modifying your workout routine to accommodate a more unpredictable sleep schedule demonstrates adaptability.

Prioritizing Self-Care: Continued self-care is crucial for sustaining radiant health beyond childbirth. This involves finding moments for personal rejuvenation, whether it's taking a short walk, enjoying a hot bath, or indulging in a hobby. By prioritizing self-care, mothers can recharge both physically and mentally, contributing to their overall well-being.

Balancing Parenting Responsibilities: Finding a balance between parenting responsibilities and personal well-being is an ongoing challenge. Establishing a support system, involving partners, family, or friends, can help distribute the load. For example, scheduling dedicated "me-time" when a partner takes over childcare duties allows for moments of self-care without neglecting parental responsibilities.

Nutritional Continuity: Maintaining a nutrient-rich diet post-pregnancy is essential for both maternal recovery and the well-being of the baby, especially if breastfeeding. Incorporating foods rich in vitamins, minerals, and antioxidants supports energy levels and overall health. Meal planning and preparation can make it easier to ensure a balanced and nourishing diet.

Mindful Parenting Practices: Applying mindfulness practices to parenting fosters a positive and harmonious environment for both parents and the child. Being present in the moment, practicing patience, and embracing the challenges with a mindful mindset contribute to a healthier parent-child relationship. For instance, incorporating short mindfulness exercises into daily routines, such as mindful breathing during diaper changes, can create moments of connection.

Strengthening Family Bonds: Family bonds play a crucial role in the post-pregnancy phase. Strengthening connections with extended family members not only provides emotional support but can also offer practical assistance. Grandparents, aunts, or uncles may contribute to childcare, allowing parents some time for self-care or couple activities.

Professional Support and Guidance: Seeking professional support, whether through postpartum therapy, lactation consultants, or parenting classes, can be invaluable. These resources offer guidance on physical and emotional well-being, helping mothers navigate the challenges of post-pregnancy life. For instance, participating in postpartum fitness classes with certified instructors can provide a safe and supportive environment for physical recovery.

Setting Realistic Goals: Establishing realistic goals post-pregnancy is crucial for avoiding unnecessary stress. Whether it's returning to work, pursuing hobbies, or achieving fitness milestones, setting achievable and gradual objectives ensures a smoother transition. Celebrating small victories, like reaching a fitness milestone or completing a personal project, contributes to a positive mindset.

Conclusion: Chapter 12 encapsulates the essence of sustaining radiant health beyond childbirth. It emphasizes the continuous nature of the wellness journey, encouraging adaptability, self-care, and a holistic approach to post-pregnancy life. By integrating these practices, mothers can not only navigate the challenges but also thrive in the rewarding experience of parenting while maintaining their own well-being. The chapter serves as a guide to embarking on the next phase of the radiant wellness journey, embracing the joys and growth that come with motherhood.